Essential Oils for Sleep and Insomnia
by Sandra Will

1. What You Will Discover

Essential Oils for Insomnia and Sleep provides information and advice enabling you to use essential oils to help ensure you get the sleep you need and restore a pleasant quality of life.

In this book you will also discover:

1. What is insomnia and what causes it

2. What are essential oils and why you should use them

3. How to use essential oils safely

4. The most powerful essential oils to help you regain sleep and regain a better quality of life

2. What is Insomnia and What Causes It?

Insomnia is the inability to sleep long enough to wake up feeling revitalized. It is surprisingly common and thought to affect around one in every three people in modern societies. It is even more common amongst the elderly.

Signs of suffering from insomnia include:

- difficulty falling asleep
- remain awake for a number of hours before falling asleep
- wake up regularly through the night
- waking up the following morning still feeling tired
- inability to sleep during
- feeling withdrawn and irritable throughout the day
- have difficulty focusing on certain tasks

For most people bouts of insomnia may come and go but in severe cases insomnia can last for several years. This is referred to as 'chronic insomnia' and can have a damaging effect on a person's quality of life, affecting their mood, ability to build relationships with friends and family and the inability to plan and concentrate on various aspects of their day-to-day lives.

Insomnia can be caused by a wide variety of factors, however, they most often fall into the following categories:

- Stress and anxiety
- Noisy, cold, bright or damp environment
- Jet lag, alcohol, caffeine and working shifts
- Depression and schizophrenia
- Heart problems and long-term pain
- Medications for epilepsy, antidepressants, steroid medication

3. What Can You Do About Insomnia?

Along with using essential oils, which we shall go into detail later on in this book, there are a range of solutions you can use to help reduce insomnia and improve the amount of sleep you are receiving:

- Set times at which you go to bed and aim to wake up
- Relax before going to bed. Taking a warm shower or bath can help greatly. You can also try relaxing music to help you unwind.
- Use blackout curtains or thick blinds to block out as much light as possible.
- Avoid consuming caffeine, nicotine, sugary drinks, and large meals and in the build up to when you want to sleep.
- Reduce the amount of electrical items you use in the hour leading up to going to bed.
- Avoid sleeping during the day.
- Write a list of your stresses and concerns along with a list of solutions to help resolve issues and anxieties which are preventing you from sleeping.

When it comes to how much sleep you need the answer is that everyone is different. However, a "normal" number of hours of sleep an adult should take each day is approximately eight hours. Children and young infants can sleep for as much as twelve hours each day.

The important aspect to remember is that an adult should receive enough sleep for them to wake up feeling revitalized and the sleep you are getting is deep and energizing.

4. What Are Essential Oils?

Essential oils are the life's blood which flow a large selection plants and flowers. They are packed with completely natural plant and flora particles, including the resin, flowers, bark, leaves, and peels. Essential oils are gathered from plants using a process of water or steam distillation or by mechanical processing. The two most common methods of using essential oils include aromatherapy and topical application. Aromatherapy involves heating an essential oil in a diffuser. This process releases the particles in the oil into the are, allowing them enter our nose canal and travel directly to the brain. Once inside the brain the particle are received by the limbic system, the area of the brain which controls our moods and emotions. Depending on the oil we use we may feel more relaxed, more motivated, or more sleepy. They can also deliver a range of health benefits, including relieving joint pain, inflammation, or digestive ailments. Topical application is a process of applying essential oils to our skin which allows the tiny particles within essential oils to pass through our skins pores and into our bloodstream. Once inside our bloodstream the particles deliver the same benefits as aromatherapy. Providing us with the same benefits as aromatherapy. Although their initial use dates back over thousands of years the popularity of essential oils has grown rapidly in recent decades, part in thanks to their easy availability thanks to the arrival of the Internet and they are now widely used as natural cleaning products, skin care products, treating pets and ward off bugs and insects from the home.

When using essential oils, it is important to remember one of the fundamental aspects of essential oils is that 'a little goes a long way.' Therefore, you only need 1-2 drops of an essential to deliver their properties. Applying too much oil to the blood can lead to blood poisoning, nausea, and headaches. Therefore, it is important to use essential oils in small doses. To apply them safely to your skin you should blend a few drops with a much larger dose of 'carrier oil'. A carrier oil is similar to an essential oil but is much safer to use and doesn't feature the highly potent chemicals found in essential oils. The most popular carrier oils include jojoba, coconut oil, and sweet almond. They are called carrier oils because they carry the essential oil safely to the skin.

5. The Most Powerful Essential Oil to Help Combat Insomnia

To help you sleep you will need an essential oil that helps you to relax and feel calm. The most effective oils are those which feature sedative properties and deep relaxing aromas. The use of herbal pillows have been used in folk medicine for hundreds of years, but it was only in the early 1990's that the sedative effects of a range of essential oils were first scientifically studied. Whereby Scientists first found evidence that essential oils could, in fact, help to promote sleep and support deep relaxation. The key components found in essential oils which promote sleep were found to be linalool and linalyl acetate, natural chemicals which help to sedate the body with little or no side effects. The following oils work best to help to treat insomnia and help you to sleep better:

Lavender

Lavender is the most popular mint based essential oil and is backed by scientific research which shows it features sleep inducing properties. Helping the mind to relieve stress and anxiety which makes it easier for people to fall asleep. You can infuse your pillow with a lavender spray or simply add one or two drops to a ball of cotton wool and leave it on the bedside table.

Roman Chamomile

Roman Chamomile features a light floral aroma which is considered one of the most relaxing and calming oils available. Simply add a few drops to a diffuser to burn the oil and release the chemicals into the air or add one to two drops to a carrier oil and rub into the soles of your feet. Both methods can be incredibly effective in helping to promote sleep.

Cedarwood

Along with featuring powerful antiseptic, anti-inflammatory, and expectorant properties, it's warm, woody aroma of Cedarwood oil is also calming and relaxing. Helping to reduce anxiety and comfort in the mind. Cedarwood also helps to bring you closer to nature and help you to discover your spirituality.

Orange

Orange essential oil is excellent at helping to reduce anxiety and help you to feel more energised and motivated. Use it throughout the day to help ward off tiredness and prevent you from taking naps during the day. Sleeping during the daytime can also lead to insomnia. Creating a vicious cycle of sleeping during the day and feeling withdrawn, anxious and stressed at night as you try to get a good nights sleep. Add a few drops to a carrier oil and rub into your chest when you wake in the morning or burn in a diffuser throughout the morning.

Valerian

One of the most popular oils to aid with sleep, Valerian promotes relaxation and sleep. It can be applied topically by blending it with a carrier oil or using aromatherapy.

6. What is Aromatherapy In Detail?

Aromatherapy is a process of burning an essential oil in a diffuser and breathing in the vapors. This process directly effects our emotions and can take place within a matter of seconds, delivering the stress relief and mood-lifting benefits of essential oils both quickly and efficiently.

Traditional diffusers combine the essential oil with water or a carrier oil to make the essential oil safer to consume. Using a 100% dosage of oil can lead to absorbing too many oil molecules, leading to potential headaches and nausea. You should also use essential oils in a well-ventilated area where you have access to fresh air and you should also use aromatherapy for less than 60 minutes each day. This is plenty of time for the natural chemicals in essential oils to go to work and deliver their benefits to the recipient.

Along with conventional diffusers which fill the entire room with an aroma you can also use modern style diffusers such as those which fit on the end of a pen, a necklace pendant or plug into a car's cigarette lighter. Along with more making personal to use these modern diffusers also to help to support our lifestyles, enabling us to absorb essential oils whether we are traveling or at work without affecting other people.

7. What Is Topical Application In Detail?

A massage is a process of manipulating the bodies soft tissues including the connective tissues, muscles, ligaments, tendons and joints. A massage can alleviate discomfort, relieve stress, and pain from the body. To create a massage oil using an essential oil you first need to blend the oil with a carrier oil. A carrier oil is far less concentrated than an essential oil making the massage oil weaker and safer to use. Because essential oils are incredibly potent and consist of powerful molecules applying them directly to the skin in large quantities can poison the bloodstream. Leading to nausea, vomiting, diarrhea, and other illnesses. It is possible to deliver a self-massage which can provide a range of health benefits including helping to treat muscle wounds, joint ache and to relieve stress.

There is a range of massage techniques which you can use and courses you can take either online or at your local college to help you develop a professional massage technique. However, the key process is to start lightly and slowly build up to more rigorous strokes. This will enable you to test the firmness of the muscle and to prepare them for more force which will help to alleviate stress for more deep-lying muscles within the body. The process of a massage also helps to promote blood circulation within the muscles and skin. It is also important to avoid large bone groups and joints. The shoulder blades and back are an excellent place to start. To help as a beginner, you can use a massaging ball or roller. Helping to spread the force you are applying while still impacting on the muscles deeply to make relieve stress and tension.

8. Using Essential Oils Safely

For the majority of people, using essential oils is completely safe. However, essential oils can also interact with other medicines, homeopathic remedies or herbal products. Making them weaker or stronger. If you do have any doubts or concerns, it is best to err on the side of caution and not to use essential oils until you have spoken to your doctor. You should also avoid using essential oils completely if you fall into any of the following categories:

- Pregnant or breastfeeding
- Taking pharmaceutical drugs or cancer treatments
- Suffer from epilepsy, fits or seizures
- Have kidney disease or liver problems

When you start using essential oils you should begin by using them in small doses, testing them on small spots of your skin to see if the oil reacts. You should also use them in a well-ventilated room and away from young children and small pets. Adults have much thicker skin than children or small pets. This results in children and small pets being more prone to poisoning, so it is important not to use aromatherapy around them. You should also wash your hands after using essential oils to ensure no residue is transferred to a child or small pet.

9. Using Pure Essential Oils

Before using essential oils, it is important to take a step back and to spend some time discussing something which many other books overlook. And that is the importance of only using pure essential oils as only pure essential oils feature the natural chemicals which directly affect our emotions and support us physically. Sadly, some essential oil producers blend in synthetic ingredients with raw essential oil harvested from the plant, weakening the potency of the natural oil to produce a larger volume of stock at a much lower price than producing 100% pure essential oil. Creating bigger profits for the producer. Along with degrading their shelf life and potentially poisoning us with man-made substances, synthetic oils offer far more limited benefits to the user than using pure essential oils, making synthetic oils almost worthless to use and dangerous. To identify the purity of an essential oil, you should always look for the word "Pure" in the description of the oil. Such as "Pure Lavender Essential Oil". You may also see the words "Natural Grown" which also denotes that the ingredients within the oil are natural and pure.

When purchasing essential oils it also important to avoid the word "fragrance", this often means that the oil will feature some form of synthetic ingredients. One of the most dangerous synthetic ingredients is Phthalates. Phthalates are used in petrochemical-derived oils and are thought to have the potential to cause damage to the liver, kidneys, and reproductive organs.

It is also important to keep essential oils safe. Keeping them stored in air sealed brown glass bottles and out of direct sunlight is the most effective method to prevent them from turning rancid and instead help them to maintain their potency. Essential oils also have a typical shelf life of seven years, so it is important to dispose of them after the expiration date on the packaging.

10. Essential Oil Blends for Insomnia

The following essential oil blends are simple to use and focus on treating insomnia:

Blend #1 for Insomnia

You will need:

2 oz	Spray Bottle
2 oz	Distilled Water
15 drops	Lavender Essential Oil
10 drops	Roman Chamomile Essential Oil

Add the ingredients to the bottle and shake well. Spray 4 or 5 dashes of the formula to your pillow.

Blend #2 for Insomnia

You will need:

2 oz	Spray Bottle
2 oz	Distilled Water
12 drops	Lavender Essential Oil
6 drops	Benzoin Resin

Add the ingredients to the bottle and shake well. Spray 4 or 5 dashes of the formula to your pillow before going to sleep. The benzoin is a sticky substance so it may build up in the nozzle to your spray bottle. Spray 4 or 5 dashes of the formula to your pillow before going to sleep.

Blend #3 for Insomnia

You will need:

An Essential Oil Diffuser
20 drops   Sweet Marjoram Essential Oil
25 drops   Lavender Essential Oil.

Blend the lavender and sweet marjoram oils together in a bowl or pestle. Add five drops of the mixture to the diffuser in the hours leading up to going to sleep.

Blend #4 for Insomnia

You will need:

2 oz   Spray Bottle
2 oz   Distilled Water
15 drops   Lavender Essential Oil
10 drops   Sweet Marjoram Essential Oil

Add the ingredients to the bottle and shake well. Spray 4 or 5 dashes of the formula to your pillow before going to sleep.

Blend #5 for Insomnia

You will need:

2 oz   Spray Bottle
2 oz   Distilled Water
15 drops   Lavender Essential Oil
5 drops   Bergamot Essential Oil

Add the ingredients to the bottle and shake well. Spray 4 or 5 dashes of the formula to your pillow before going to sleep.

Blend #6 for Insomnia

You will need:

8 drops	Roman Chamomile
4 drops	Clary Sage
4 drops	Bergamot

Add three drops of the mixture to a tissue and place underneath the pillow or on the bedside table.

Blend #7 for Insomnia

You will need:

8 drops	Roman Chamomile
4 drops	Clary Sage
4 drops	Bergamot

Add three drops of the mixture to a tissue and place underneath the pillow or on the bedside table.

Blend #8 for Insomnia

You will need:

2 oz	Spray Bottle
2 oz	Distilled Water
10 drops	Roman Chamomile
2 drops	Lemon Essential Oil

Add the ingredients to the bottle and shake well. Spray 4 or 5 dashes of the formula to your pillow before going to sleep. Too much lemon and the scent will be too sweet but two drops will help to make the mixture more pleasant.

Blend #9 for Insomnia

You will need:

| 2 oz | Spray Bottle |

2 oz	Distilled Water
10 drops	Vetiver
10 drops	Mandarin Essential Oil

Add the ingredients to the bottle and shake well. Spray 4 or 5 dashes of the formula to your pillow before going to sleep. This will provide a balanced and warm fragrance to fall asleep to.

Blend #10 for Insomnia

You will need:

An Essential Oil Diffuser
10 drops	Roman Chamomile
30 drops	Lavender Essential Oil

Blend the oils together in a small bowl or pestle. Add five drops of the mixture to the diffuser and burn before going to sleep.

11. Creating a Soothing Environment

Giving our senses as much peace and freedom from the stresses around is essential to relax and unwind. A process that is vital to helping us to sleep better when we need to. One of the most effective methods to give our senses an opportunity to relax is to establish an environment that is naturally soothing and allows us to relieve stress.

Lighting

If you are indoors, you need to create a relaxing and soothing level of lighting using as much natural light as possible. Meditating in a brightly lit room makes it difficult to relax and unwind as our sense of sight is disrupted by the strong light, making it harder for us to relax and reduce stress. The best place to meditate is outside, bringing you closer to nature and fresh air.

Noise

Finding a peaceful and quiet place is also vital to both yoga and meditation. Scheduling your time and letting other people around you know that this is your period of meditation will allow you to create an environment which is free from disruption, enabling you to find mental clarity without any distraction or disturbance. You may also want to use a recording of natural sounds such as birds tweeting or the sound of sea waves crashing together.

Smell

The aroma of essential oil burnt in a diffuser is the most powerful and effective method of helping the mind to relax and to enjoy meditation or yoga. To create a clean smell you may want to meditate as far away from the kitchen as possible. Any lingering aromas from fried onions or the smell of spicy food will make it more difficult to relax and meditate. You should also avoid meditating in a room with artificial fragrances including air fresheners. They not only feature chemicals but are entirely unnecessary. Aromatherapy provides an aroma which is full of natural compounds which uplift our emotions and reduce stress.

Clutter

A cluttered space is a cluttered mind, so it is important to try and meditate somewhere you have room to move and is safe. Being outside in a park or even on the beach are perfect places to meditate and connect with nature.

Having a soothing environment in which you can meditate or practice yoga in is essential in enabling you discover mental clarity and improve your life.

12. Benefits of Yoga and Meditation

A number of scientific studies have also identified how yoga and meditation can also be used to relieve stress and help us to unwind. Helping us to sleep better at night. Examples of the findings include:

1. Increased Concentration

When we meditate or practice yoga, we are in essence exercising our brain, forcing it to concentrate on finding peace and mindfulness. Using the control of our breath and focusing our mind on a single emotion increases our level of concentration to strengthen our level of mental clarity and happiness. However, concentrating our mind on one single thought or one single part of our body is notoriously difficult to achieve and can take many hours of practice to master. This level of practice and mastery enables us to develop the skill to focus our mind more sharply and to avoid distraction. Helping us to concentrate better on our work or personal objectives. Allowing us to avoid stress by completing the things we need to maintain a quality of life which makes us happy.

2. Meditation Relieves Stress

Meditation requires the mind to enter a phase of deep relaxation. Bringing stress to the surface of our thoughts and expelling it out of our bodies as we control our breath. Relieving stress allows us to create space in our mind, allowing us to think through solutions to the problems in our lives. Practicing yoga also encourages us to stretch our muscles and release built up tension and cramp which can weigh down on our body and lead to stress.

3. Meditation Can Treat Depression

Many of us will experience some form of depression at some point in our lives. However, using meditation to relieve stress and bring tranquility into our lives is now considered a powerful method to reduce the prospect of becoming depressed. Health authorities throughout the world including in Britain are beginning to prescribe courses in meditation to help people to recover from the mental illness of depression. If you believe you are suffering from depression, it is important to seek help from your doctor. However, using meditation and yoga could be the answer many people are looking for to improve their mental health and quality of life.

4. Boosts Our Immune System

External factors can alter our immune system. For example, people who regularly do cardiovascular exercise or practice yoga tend to have stronger immune systems compared to people who tend to lead more sedentary lifestyles. It has also been recognized in recent studies that people who regularly practice meditation also have stronger immune systems. Enabling people who practice meditation and yoga to live longer and have a better quality of life.

13. Stress Management

As we discussed previously, stress is one of the most common factors which can prevent us from gaining the sleep that we need. Stress is a spiral that ratchets itself up as we move deeper into complex situations involving factors outside of our control. When we feel emotionally stressed and physically tired, we tend to produce unhealthy toxins in our bodies. Using essential oils in combination with meditation enables us to lower these toxins, relieve stress and improve our overall health. When our bodies begin to relax, we reduce the side effects of stress which include high blood pressure, aches, insomnia, headaches, and heart conditions. Essential oils also add nutrients that were part of the original plant. These nutrients cleanse our bodies, relax our mind and support our overall health.

There are other techniques which can reduce stress including the use of humor, physical exercise, hydration, power sleeping or distancing yourself from the stress. However, meditation and yoga provide a highly effective method of reducing stress and creating a level of mental clarity which enables us to both avoid stress and to use the mental clarity to find solutions and answers to the problems facing us. Allowing us to boost our level of self-confidence and create a positive outcome for any event we may face. Essential oils can be used to reduce stress and calm the mind. Allowing you to enter a calm and relaxed mental state more quickly. By being able to create mental clarity within our mind, we are also able to identify the mistakes we have made along with changes we could make to live better and happier lives. Having a clear mind is vital for us to prosper and remain healthy. You can achieve this by incorporating essential oils with meditation or yoga.

14. Essential Oils for Mental Clarity

Essential oils also provide a powerful and completely natural resource to help mind discover mental clarity. A key figure which helps us to focus on solutions to the problems which are preventing us from sleeping well at night and to also develop self-confidence and self-esteem.

The following essential oils are incredibly useful at providing specific support to help us find mental clarity:

Bergamot features a clean, refreshing fragrance which relieves anxiety and lifts our emotional mood. Add one or two drops to a personal inhaler or ball of cotton wool to inhale.

Ylang Ylang is widely used in floral perfumes and aromatherapy. It's rich floral aroma helps to expel negative emotions, flooding the mind with thoughts of nature and calmness. It's aroma also helps to boost spirituality and encourage the mind to focus on positive emotions.

Melissa, or lemon balm, has been used for thousands of years to help treat a variety of ailments including nervous disorders and stress. However, it also features anxiolytic properties which help to balance emotions and uplift mood. Use occasionally for a number of weeks to help instill a more positive outlook on life.

Sandalwood is one of the most potent oils at stimulating the brain's limbic system to help stabilize emotions and relieve anxiety.

Having skills and hobbies in our life is also vital to building confidence and self-esteem. Developing a strong understanding of essential oils is a simple way to develop skills and a hobby that we enjoy, gives us pleasure and relieves stress. Practicing essential oils also provides us with evidence to our inner self that we can achieve things in life. Creating a foundation on which we can build long-term self-confidence and self-esteem.

The uplifting aroma of essential oils can also be used to boost creativity and stimulate the mind into taking action to develop completely new skill and expertise. Using essential oils to boost confidence also enables us to be more productive, allowing us to focus on achieving our goals and overcome our fears without worrying or being to scared to take action.

Using essential oils to motivate and make us feel more alert also changes our body language. Making us appear more active and confident around other people. Whether we like it or not, our body language plays a massive role in the way other people treat us. Therefore, having a positive and outgoing body language makes other people comfortable around us. Meeting people who judge us as being someone who is alert and confident also helps to create a positive cycle of proving to ourselves that we can be confident and outgoing. Building strong relationships with other people can also help to build self-esteem and foundations to build the sort of life we want.

Having a passion and skill for essential oils is also something you can share with your friends and family. Having something positive in your life to discuss with other people is an incredibility effective method to building confidence. Each time you talk to other people about your interests and passions you are enforcing your subconscious mind that you do have skills and knowledge. Therefore, essential oils can play a significant role in building positive cycles in our lives which can develop firm foundations for confidence and self-esteem.

Useful Website Addresses

Along with www.esseentialoilsbookclub.com you can also use the following resources to learn more about essential oils:

http://www.beoa.co.uk – British Essential Oil Association

https://www.naha.org - National Association for Holistic Aromatherapy (USA)

http://airase.com - Association for the International Research of Aromatic Science and Education

http://www.a-t-c.org.uk – Aromatherapy Trade Council

http://efeo-org.org - European Federation of Essential Oils

http://www.ifaroma.org - International Federation of Aromatherapists

http://www.eoai.in - Essential oil association of India

http://www.thesma.org - The Association for Soft Tissue Therapists

http://www.iaim.org.uk - International Association of Infant Massage

http://www.alliance-aromatherapists.org - Alliance of International Aromatherapists

Clearing the Air: Smoking Cessation Services in the UK and their Benefits to Society

About the author

Seán O'Connor is a dedicated and compassionate professional, who has made significant contributions to the field of smoking cessation services within the United Kingdom. With a deep-rooted passion for public health and a wealth of experience as a Smoking Cessation Advisor at Manchester Public Health, Seán has been instrumental in guiding individuals towards a smoke-free life, one step at a time.

Having served as a Smoking Cessation Advisor within the esteemed framework of the National Health Service (NHS), the UK's renowned public health service, Seán honed their specialist skills in providing invaluable advice and support to those grappling with nicotine addiction. Through group interventions and one-to-one interactions, Seán demonstrated an unwavering commitment to assessing clients' motivation and readiness to quit, recognizing the multifaceted aspects of nicotine addiction, and guiding them through the challenging process of achieving freedom from tobacco.

During their tenure as a Smoking Cessation Advisor, Seán was an integral part of the local community in Manchester, utilizing their expertise to create a supportive and empowering environment for individuals seeking to break free from the shackles of smoking.

Their dedication to understanding the intricacies of nicotine addiction and their unwavering support for clients has earned them a reputation as a trusted ally and a beacon of hope in the battle against tobacco.

Now, Seán brings their wealth of knowledge and experience to the forefront with their book, "Clearing the Air: Smoking Cessation Services in the UK and their Benefits to Society." Drawing upon their first-hand experiences as a Smoking Cessation Advisor, Seán delves into the profound impact of comprehensive cessation services on individuals and society as a whole. Through their insightful exploration of the challenges, triumphs, and the societal significance of smoking cessation, Seán seeks to enlighten and inspire readers to embark on a journey toward a healthier, smoke-free future.

With their expertise and unwavering dedication, Seán aims to bridge the gap between knowledge and action, fostering a greater understanding of the benefits of smoking cessation services in the UK. Through their book, Seán invites readers to join them in advocating for a smoke-free society, where the air we breathe is clean and the collective well-being of communities is nurtured.

"Clearing the Air" stands as a testament to Seán's tireless efforts, offering readers an illuminating perspective on the transformative power of smoking cessation services and the profound benefits they bring to individuals and society alike.